Dementia

what every carer needs to know

by

Bill King

for my wife

© Bill King 2022
(This version published June 2022)

Reviews

This latest book is a masterpiece of invaluable information and advice. It covers every feature of this terrible disease but not only that, it offers profound help and understanding of the needs of the Carer especially after the grim decision made in putting one's loved one into a Care Home when the guilt, the loneliness, and the raft of emotions besiege one.

The writer's words resonated regarding the need for the Carer to look after themselves as best they can and to seek the help they will so desperately need, be it practical or emotional. Every aspect is covered. Every practicality. Every likely emotion. This sharing of this information is truly to be admired. The word invaluable I use again. (Margaret Holman)

Reviews of Bill King's previous book:
Parkinsons – the slippery slope into dementia

I found your book interesting, engaging, entertaining, and at times very moving. What made it particularly poignant is the fact that I do of course know both you and your wife personally, and although you hid her identity I could clearly recognise the person that I knew so well.

I am sure the written account only gives a flavour of everything you have had to go through, and all the pain that you suffered at seeing a loved one deteriorate in this way. Being able to put all this down on paper will, I'm sure, be of considerable benefit to others who might find themselves in this situation. (Murdo Fraser, MSP)

Most of us think we understand Parkinsons but in reality we don't have a clue, unless you live with a family member and have to deal with everything it throws at you, every single day, as you watch your loved one change in front of your eyes.

This is not an easy read in places and I found it emotionally challenging. I felt I was being re-educated, to my shame, as I was one of those who wasn't aware of or didn't understand the obstacles and difficulties 'Bill King' has had to contend with as he lovingly cared for his wife.

None of us knows what lies in store for us, and perhaps that is for the best in some ways, but this book brings to the fore love and despair in equal amounts. I would have no hesitation in recommending you buy it and let others know about it. (Provost Dennis Melloy, Perth and Kinross)

I read the book in two sittings which maybe gives you an indication of how interesting I found it. It certainly opened my eyes more to the challenges carers face trying to deal with a loved one coping with this awful illness and it just makes me more determined to try and do more. (Raymond Jamieson, Carers Hub Manager, PKAVS)

I have just finished reading your book. Thank you for allowing me to share your experience. Having worked in a care home followed by a spell in home care, I have witnessed this scenario many times, also personally, with each of the main carers being brought into a hopeless situation.
This has been a sensitive, touching read and an experience echoed by millions throughout the land, but you have given a little light relief and understanding to the harsh reality and the book gives a true insight to make others feel they are not alone. (LMG)

You have given your wife love by the bucket load. It is clear that it has been a love match. Will she remember this? Who knows, but you will know this and I sincerely hope it will eventually bring you comfort.

In the greatest way you have bared your soul as well as giving information of great value. I cannot tell you how impressed I am with the content. For me it strikes the perfect note. It is informative, touching and with the degree of humour necessary. I thought you expressed yourself very well. I am sure it will resonate with many readers. (MH)

(Note: PKAVS = Perth and Kinross Association of Voluntary Service.)

Table of contents

Two possible scenarios from the past 8
A clutch of quotes – some even positive...9
Author's note..11

Part one – Setting the scene 13

Chapter one – Introduction 15
Chapter two – Patient-centred treatment......................................20

Part two – Doing the groundwork 23

Chapter three – Practical matters 25
    (a) Power of attorney (POA) 26
    (b) Drawing up a will..27
    (c) A living will 27
    (d) Getting professional care 27
    (e) Blue badge..28
    (f) Money and savings 28
    (g) Make a record of bank, etc, passwords and other details 29
    (h) Practical purchases 29
    (i) Dehydration 30
    (j) Medication 30
    (j) Family history 31
    (k) Keeping a journal 31
Chapter four – A dementia-friendly home 33
    (a) Flooring 34
    (b) Grab handles 34
    (c) Local authority supplies 35
    (d) Lifts and stair lifts 35
    (e) Bath and shower 36
    (f) Commode..36
    (g) User-friendly doors 36
    (h) Bedtime 38
    (i) Seating 39

    (j) Alexa and friends 40
    (k) Outside the building 40
    (l) Wheelchairs and other equipment..................................40
    (m) Personal Alarms 41
    (n) Helping hands 41
Chapter five – Being prepared as a carer 43
Chapter six – General advice in advance 47
    (a) Don't take it personally. 48
    (b) Do not boss or order your loved one about. 48
        Mental issues...50
    (a) Communication and distraction. 50
    (b) Short-term memory loss..50
    (c) compulsive/repetitive behaviour 51
Chapter seven – Reacting as a carer...55
    (a) The value of 'active listening'...55
    (b) Unequal relationship 55
    (c) Slow down..56
    (d) When the sun goes down 56
    (e) Trust your own judgment 57
Chapter eight – Foot in mouth 59
    (a) Talking about the past 59
    (b) Right and wrong..61
    (c) Hallucinations 61
    (d) I wonder how so and so is? 62
    (e) Responding to paranoia 62
Chapter nine – Coping with dementia..63
    (a) What's the time? What day is it? 63
    (b) loss of balance...64
    (c) wandering..65
    (d) unwillingness to take medication 66
    (e) disturbed sleep patterns 66
    (f) cognitive issues..66
    (g) The five senses 67
        Smell 67
        Hearing..67
        Vision 68

Touch	68
Taste	69
Summary	69
(h) Colours and their problems	69
(i) Don't contradict	69
(j) The incomplete sentence	70
(k) urinary or double incontinence	71
Chapter ten – Coping with dementia (continued)	72
(a) Problems with food	72
(b) retail issues	73
(c) psychosis (delirium or UTI related)	74
(d) The need to go into a care home	74
Chapter eleven – Visiting your loved one	75
Part three – Caring for the carer	79
Chapter twelve – Who needs care?	81
Chapter thirteen – Educating carers	83
Chapter fourteen – Facing 'anticipatory grief'	85
Endpiece	91
Sources	93
Books	93
Films	94
Websites	95
A clutch of quotes to end with	96

Author's note

My name has been rebadged with a pseudonym again to protect the identity of my family, and my wife's name has also been altered to Rusalka.

You will note that I omit the apostrophe from Parkinsons – it is becoming more usual to see this change and I feel it makes the word look better on the page, especially when used in isolation.

I make no apologies for being a bit repetitious in what follows. Some of what I have to say inevitably overlaps a little with my previous book, and if you wish to consult specific subsections of the text, I shall repeat bits of relevant advice to avoid your having to scrabble round the book for information.

As with the *Parkinsons* book, which is also available on Amazon, all proceeds go to local dementia charities.

Once again I offer my thanks to my indefatigable duo of main beta testers/proof readers, Liz Gordon and Margaret Holman and my new recruit Libby Melloy. Any remaining errors are of my own making.

I have posted a short introductory video about the book on YouTube, which can be most easily visited by going to my website www.locheesoft.com and clicking on the link on the home page. There is also a video available for *Parkinsons – the slippery slope to dementia*.

Two possible scenarios from the past

First scenario: you are recovering from a broken leg in a hospital ward and your nurse asks you to take a shower. 'No, thank you,' you reply, stating that you are in pain, tired and would rather wash later. No problem there. The nurse goes off and leaves you to your own devices.

Second scenario: you are in the dementia section of a care home. 'Time for a shower,' states one of the staff assertively. 'No, thank you,' you reply, complaining that you are tired and in pain, and would rather wash later. It takes three or four staff to carry you forcibly to the shower, undress you and wash you. You are accused of being uncooperative and wilful.

Such was a perhaps extreme example of the long-established medical model of dementia, with the patient regarded as an insentient being with little or no human worth. The pioneering medics who have been seeking to create a new and more humane approach are still engaged in a struggle with outmoded notions – and, to be honest, much public sentiment – which are deeply entrenched.

The battle to ensure that the person with dementia is treated as a human being with positive qualities, not a collection of symptoms to be managed as they decline and rapidly lose their last shreds of humanity, is far from over, especially among the public at large. In their book, Rahmen and Howard (see bibliography) insist: 'Rather than fitting the person to the services, services should fit the person.' Sometimes that assertion still seems to echo my wishful thinking about medical interventions generally: 'The patient will see you now, doctor.' Some chance...

A clutch of quotes – some even positive

You are not your illness. You have an individual story to tell. Staying yourself is part of the battle. – Julian Seifter

Solitude is fine but you need someone to tell that solitude is fine. – Honoré de Balzac.

The need for human intimacy for most people lasts until the end of their life. – Kuhn.

It's far better to be unhappy alone than unhappy with someone. – Marilyn Monroe.

Two possibilities exist: either we are alone in the Universe or we are not. Both are equally terrifying. – Arthur C. Clarke.

Loneliness is the poverty of self; solitude is the richness of self. – Mary Sarton.

They say isolation drives you crazy. Sure it does – when you can't get enough of it. – Anneli Rufus.

We live as we dream – alone. – Joseph Conrad.

A season of loneliness and isolation is when the caterpillar gets its wings. – Mandy Hale.

If you think education is expensive, try ignorance. – Robert Orton.

One who is established in the self feels no loneliness. – Ravi Shankar.

A test of a people is how it behaves toward the old. It is easy to love children. But the affection and care for the old, the incurable, the helpless are the true goldmines of a culture. – Abraham Joshua Heschel.

We don't stop playing because we grow old; we grow old because we stop playing. – George Bernard Shaw.

Ask the young, they know everything. – French Proverb.

My mother is going to have to stop lying about her age because pretty soon I'm going to be older than she is. – Tripp Evan.

You know you are getting old when the candles cost more than the cake. – Bob Hope.

People who have dementia, for whom the life of the emotion is often intense, and without the ordinary forms of inhibition, may have something important to teach the rest of mankind. – Tom Kitwood.

People, even more than things, have to be restored, renewed, revived, reclaimed, and redeemed. Never throw out anyone. – Audrey Hepburn.

Do you want to meet the love of your life? Look in the mirror. – Byron Katie.

What lies behind you and what lies in front of you, pales in comparison to what lies inside of you. – Ralph Waldo Emerson.

A word of encouragement during a failure is worth more than an hour of praise after success. – Anonymous.

No one can make you feel inferior without your consent. – Eleanor Roosevelt.

Our greatest glory is not in never falling, but in rising every time we fall. – Confucius.

(There are more quotes lurking at the end of this book.)

Part one – Setting the scene

Chapter one – Introduction

The idea for this book came to me soon after I had finished *Parkinsons – the slippery slope to dementia*, when it dawned on me that I had failed to tell the whole story of the carer's needs. In fact, I had left out of the equation two vital areas of concern to the carer, which is not surprising, as no one else seems to have given them much credence.

Dementia is an illness recognised by the medical professionals and is therefore treated and managed as best they can given the lack of a cure and the residual prejudices of the medical model of the patient. However, being a carer has no medical status at all, and despite the invaluable role they play, they have been sorely neglected in two respects in particular.

Of course (people will say) carers receive a lot of support: financial, carers' groups, one-to one-counselling, and so on, but the one vital thing they are not given by way of properly organised good practice is professionally sound advanced and suitably detailed information of what to expect and how to deal with it as a carer. Over the years, I found myself firefighting, whereas fire prevention would have been preferable – and potentially less damaging, to say the least.

That was one of the factors which most distressed me when I was a full-time carer, the feeling that I was always playing catch-up, walking blindfolded into unfamiliar territory with no means of knowing how to cope, or of recognising if my efforts in so doing were potentially counterproductive or even harmful to my loved one. Only afterwards did I tend to find out the information which should have been available to me well before the event.

As I have told the professionals repeatedly, I am flying on a wing and a prayer; I have not done this before, and on top of that, I have not been given the tools to cope with the crises large and small which may arise in the process of caring for my loved one. I am not only making unnecessary mistakes, I am also in danger of compounding faults which draw on outdated and mistaken attitudes to mental impairment, and which could well have a negative impact on the person being cared for – and a knock-on effect on the overstretched carer, too.

If carers were by right offered the opportunity to be trained in advance to deal with everything from eating issues to full-blown psychoses, I would have been able to respond to them more appropriately and with less emotional cost to us both. And my second area of concern is: no one ever should say to the carer whose loved one has gone into a care home: 'Job done. You can relax now.'

That is a situation which I know personally can be even more traumatic than full-time personal caring was, and for which support and advance information is also sadly lacking. I did not have the tools to learn how to cope with this 'anticipatory grief' or 'living bereavement' of now living alone, and I continue to need appropriate information and support when I visit my wife and attempt to keep up with how to cope with her shifting and deteriorating condition.

The Alzheimer's Society website expresses my feelings admirably with these words:

> For some carers, anticipatory grief can be even harder to deal with than the grief they feel after the person has died. For some people, anticipatory grief may lead to depression. It can help to talk about these feelings while you are still caring for the person with dementia.

I hope I have thus far made the outline of a case for making the carer a key and appropriately well-informed person in the vital process of coping with a loved one in their challenging and ever-developing situation, and for giving the person they are caring for the life opportunities they deserve.

However, unlike many politicians I could name, but won't, I am not content to stand on the sidelines moaning about an undesirable situation. I am actually doing something about it. That's what this book is all about.

I know there is plenty of good information out there – but taking the time to chase it all down is of little consolation for anyone daunted by the prospect of trawling across the internet and diving into in the plethora of books on dementia, some of them highly technical in their language. In any event, you are far from sure where to look until a problem has actually arisen, and then you are too busy trying to cope with it to take time out looking.

So what I am offering here is a one-stop shop, as it were, for you to do two things: to have advanced notice of the more common problems that can arise when caring for someone with dementia, and secondly, as soon as a particular problem does emerge, you can return to these pages to remind yourself of the appropriate actions to take.

Not much is entirely original, and I can't cover every possibility, but the key point is that I have done all the spadework and assembled a whole raft of key information in one place for you. I hope what follows will be a significant means of support and advice to assist you in what I know will be a huge and growing challenge which will rapidly come to consume most of your waking hours.

It's imperfect, but I'm reminded of the old Chinese proverb, which states that 'A journey of a thousand miles begins with a single step'. Someone has to have a go, and that someone usually gets a lot of flak for so doing, but, hey, I am a glutton for punishment.

There is one other central issue I'd like to address from the outset, at the risk of repeating myself a little. There has indeed been a hugely welcome shift over recent years from the old 'medical model' of the dementia patient to a 'patient-centred' approach, which sounds technical but is in fact absolutely crucial for people with dementia.

Put crudely, there used to be a policy of treating dementia patients as lesser humans, or even non-humans whose cognitive powers had been more or less switched off and who needed to be pushed to one side and managed in controlled environments where they could quietly fade away and be allowed to die.

This was a case of fitting the patient to the system, whereas nowadays best practice is to do exactly the reverse: to regard the person with dementia primarily as a human being with faculties which may be diminished, but a person none the less, who should be respected and treated like any other person with an illness. So now the old outmoded notions are stood on their head and the system is there to fit to the patient.

One neat example of this is the large aspirational sign on the wall near the entrance to Rusalka's own care home. It reads: 'Our residents don't live in our workspace, we work in their home.'

One reason I am stressing this is that the wider public perception of dementia can – and often still does – take the form of regarding patients as more or less brain dead, no longer human at all, lifeless from the neck up. That sounds brutal, but these misconceptions partly stem, I believe, from a visceral fear of dementia, a disease for which there is as yet no known cure, and towards which we are in danger of heading ourselves.

In recent years, life expectancy has extended way beyond past aspirations, bringing with it a range of degenerative diseases such as dementia which medical science still has no means of reversing. For this reason, one commentator has described dementia as a Cinderella disease.

Let's get that other common prejudice out of the way. Dementia is not exclusively about rows of beds filled with doubly incontinent old folk who have lost their minds and, though they don't know it, are lying there just waiting to die. Nor is it inevitably about people 'losing their mind'. Some people can function pretty well with the disease, whilst for others the prognosis is less happy.

Wendy Miller, a remarkable lady who was in senior management in the NHS, contracted dementia and yet wrote two important and emotionally charged books charting her deteriorating condition. I urge you to beg, borrow, buy or otherwise acquire a copy of her publications (see the bibliography at the end of this book), and do purchase a packet of Kleenex before reading (other tissue products are available). Make that two packets.

Chapter two – Patient-centred treatment

You may wonder why I've found it necessary to put yet more words together, especially now since my wife has entered full-time care, because, you might be tempted to think, that's it, your caring days are over, and now you can rest on your laurels.

I'm reminded of that famous TV Saturday night programme in the old black and white days known by its initials TW3, when Millicent Martin sang the opening patter song: 'That was the week that was, / It's over, let it go'. The trouble with being a carer is that even though the hard grind of full-time care may have come to an end, the problems not only linger on but they can become much more intense, and you can't simply let them go.

There appears to be an assumption amongst medical and care professionals that when the loved one goes into a care home, that's it as far as the carer is concerned. As was claimed so wrongly about the end of the Iraq war: 'Mission accomplished!' Well, it isn't. The carer needs ongoing support and also help in recognising the more advanced symptoms of dementia and how to cope with them.

The caring process is far from over, and the carer can, with a reasonable understanding of the likely symptoms of intensifying dementia, be of great value in comforting and supporting the care home resident, and he or she can gain a sense of satisfaction that they are acting in their loved one's very best interests.

I am not making any special claims for what I have put together here, except that there is a world of information out there which we are not routinely given awareness of, which can improve your dealings with the person you are caring for and increase your awareness of the processes which they are going through. Ignorance breeds fear and misapprehensions; knowledge shines a light into the darkness.

Dementia is such a varied beast which does not yield to a scattergun approach. There isn't even a convenient 'dementia gene' lurking in our DNA. It's a highly complex set of possibilities which can often be challenging to diagnose.

I am reminded of the oft-repeated cartoon of the drunk swaying uncertainly next to a lamp post late at night. A policeman comes up to him and asks what he is doing. 'I've lost my keys,' he slurs. 'You lost them under this streetlamp?' demands the officer. 'No, but it's brighter here so that's where I am looking.'

If it has a name, like dementia, it can exist as a pathological phenomenon, even though it is such a hugely complex illness with a wide range of variations. And it can be researched and treated, even if such treatments are currently of a purely palliative nature, as there is currently no cure in sight for it. There is little evidence that purely physical aberrations cause it:

> There is a sense in which genes do not 'cause' anything; they are simply a background on which other causes operate. (Kitwood, p 29)

There is another significant contributory factor in dementia which had not really struck home until I read more about it, namely, that a modern liberal society like the one in which we all live (although the 'liberal' bit is currently being challenged by the woke folk and other factors) is not particularly nimble when it comes to dealing with feelings, emotions and all that side of life.

In fact, it has for centuries been unsympathetic, to put it mildly, towards those with physical or mental deficiencies or other deviations from the norm. In that kind of situation, the three most unhelpful but frequently used words in the English language for someone in a bad situation are: 'Pull yourself together'.

It is highly important that people with dementia should be regarded as human beings like the rest of us, but with distinctive variations in their functioning. In a damning criticism of our society, Kitwood stresses that 'the process of dementia is also the story of a tragic inadequacy in our general way of life'.

It is equally vital that carers should be given the tools to perform their voluntary functions more effectively and derive greater satisfaction from their lives of relentless dedication. So in what follows, you will find not only help in caring for your loved one, you need also to know how to care for yourself. You have to be mentally and physically capable of looking after your loved one. There is no point in both of you collapsing and being in need of support.

Part two – Doing the groundwork

Chapter three – Practical matters

Now I get down to brass tacks and focus on the central purpose of this book, a list of issues which may (and in many cases, will) arise when caring for someone with dementia. I begin with a consideration of the practical steps you should consider in the early stages of the illness. I make no apologies for overlapping slightly with some of my observations in the predecessor to this book.

There are quite a few central issues which you must address, even though the early months – and in many cases, years – of caring may seem to be relatively unstressful and the symptoms too lacking in severity to be any great cause for concern. Now, though, is the time to act, and any delay will cause you quite a bit of bother when the need arises to take more serious steps.

I personally was far from happy being in a developing situation when I was playing catchup all the time. For example, when my wife was, so I thought, gradually deteriorating through Parkinsons, I was not aware of the cruel impact of psychoses on her, first hearing after the event that these were, to quote the consultant psychiatrist, 'classic manifestations' of Parkinsons. The same applied to the shift from Parkinsons to dementia.

It reminds me of the Scouts (and Guides) motto: Be Prepared. When asked what one was supposed to be prepared for, Baden Powell, the movement's founder, replied that it means 'being in a state of readiness in mind and body to do your duty'. That's just about right. The trouble for carers has been that you can't be prepared for some eventuality if you don't know it is likely to happen, and that's precisely why I am writing this book, to make sure you know what's coming down the road towards you.

So I begin with some purely practical advice, much of which should be followed as soon as possible after diagnosis.

(a) Power of attorney (POA)

You should go for POAs, as they will make life a great deal easier for you when one of you is regarded not to have mental capacity. They should be drawn up between you as soon as possible. If you don't, you can find yourself in a pickle if you have a joint account. Banks or building societies can decide how far you can access it. You will have to go to the court for decisions to be made and that can cost a lot in time and money.

There are any number of other issues which will arise if you do not have POA, and do ensure that it covers both health and welfare, and also financial matters. By the way, the word 'attorney' here does not refer to the American usage meaning 'lawyer'. It is intended to describe the role of a person acting on behalf of another.

For further information, try one or all of these websites:

1. www.gov.uk/power-of-attorney

2. mind.org.uk and type in their search box 'lasting power of attorney'.

3. www.citizensadvice.org.uk

Ensure you are on the right part of the website of number 3, depending on where in the UK you seek help. You will find loads of information and advice on everything including finance. You can of course also talk to the CAB, now rebadged as citizens advice in trendy lower case.

You can also create your own POA, and there are several books on the market which aspire to do just that. If you can afford it or if you can get funding to help, a visit to a solicitor is by far the best approach.

It is also useful to name an alternate, if both of you succumb to a disabling illness.

(b) Drawing up a will
While you are at the solicitor's you should ensure that you have both made wills. This is particularly important if just one of you owns the property you live in, and you wish to continue to live there even if you have no title to do so.

(c) A living will
If you are so minded, a so-called living will is also an option. The general purpose of such wills is to state that you do not wish to be resuscitated when certain conditions are fulfilled. You will probably come across the acronym DNR, which means 'do not resuscitate'.

Both wills and living wills can be drawn up without the aid of a solicitor, but my advice is that such an approach is a false economy, as your solicitor will be aware of all the traps and pitfalls that can occur with wills. You will not be, believe me.

(d) Getting professional care
Advice on how to claim for a Personal Independence Payment (PIP) can be found at www.gov.uk/pip/how-to-claim. With a high level of PIP, you can make use of the Motability scheme to acquire a vehicle to allow you freedom of movement.

The choice of vehicles is quite huge, and you should be aware that some require an additional down payment on your part. Motability can also assist in the adaptation of suitable vehicles in providing a hoist for a wheelchair, special changes to the controls for severely disabled drivers, and so forth.

The scheme allows you appoint a couple of named drivers and additional drivers for one off use. It is not means tested. You normally keep a vehicle from new for three years, then change the vehicle.

Do not abuse this excellent scheme. If you are caught out misusing the system, you can lose the vehicle.

Also, do be aware of the fact that if your loved one becomes a resident in a nursing home, the PIP ceases, leaving you as a carer with decisions to make regarding personal purchase of a vehicle to visit your loved one if no public transport is readily available.

(e) Blue badge
Apply to the local authority for a blue badge, enabling you if your loved one qualifies to park in disabled bays and elsewhere, too, depending on local arrangements.

(f) Money and savings
When your loved one is first diagnosed, the prospect of moving them into residential care seems remote indeed, but forward financial planning could save you some real problems further down the line, and here your solicitor will be of help too.

I refer in particular to the cost of the home and who pays. This falls into two parts. The loved one's pension, minus around £30 at the time of writing for personal weekly needs, is gobbled up by the local authority. In addition, if they are deemed to have savings above a certain level, they will be required to pay for some or all of the cost of care, which can be around £1,000 per week.

The amount of savings can be quite modest before such contributions kick in, and you should be aware of problems that might arise when you move funds out of your own savings. The penny-pinchers assessing you may tend to regard large transfers of funds as a deliberate attempt to reduce your savings below a particular threshold.

My advice is to do what I did with our local authority assessment team in mind, and that is to put together an aide-memoire listing current and deposit accounts, as well as other savings and capital, and explaining why largish chunks of money are moved around, for example, if you take out a funeral arrangements scheme for both of you, for or essential house repairs which need to be paid for.

If you are an owner occupier, a lifetime mortgage is well worth considering, as long as you are aware of its implications for inheritance. In other words, the interest can build up quite a lot, and that will reduce the amount some family members might be expecting to benefit from.

Carer's allowance can also be applied for in some circumstances.

(g) Make a record of bank, etc, passwords and other details
Over the years, Rusalka and I entered into a blank notebook – which we divided into sections from A to Z – the names and numbers of our bank accounts, and all the passwords and phone numbers which we used and changed as time went by.

This has proved a godsend for me, especially in relation to the accounts my wife set up. Even with Power of Attorney, I still need to respond to security questions like 'Which school did your wife first attend?', and 'What is her mother's maiden name?' (In our case, that was an unpronounceable string of letters transcribed from Ukrainian into English.)

I suggest that you locate the entries in your book according to the name of the company or organisation you are using: T for Tesco, N for Nationwide, and so on. Be consistent with that, otherwise you can create unnecessary confusion. For example, locating all Apple products under A is far easier than remembering if you saved them under iPad, Mac, Watch and so forth.

(h) Practical purchases
As your loved one deteriorates, there are many additional burdens you will have to take on, organising and administering medication, for example, and one important aspect is to ensure that they are well stocked with toothpaste, shower gel, and so forth.

Make certain that their spectacles are in working order and not smudged by make up or grubby hands. Hearing aid batteries may need attention, and the list goes on, varying greatly from one person to the next.

(i) Dehydration

Another practical matter demanding your attention is liquid intake. Ensure that there are bottles of water strategically located round the house, and that your loved one drinks regularly from them.

Not doing so is a result of forgetfulness, but it can have quite serious health implications.

(j) Medication

To say that this can be a contentious issue is the understatement of the century. I've had more trouble with this than any other practical matter, and I urge you to get and keep a grip on the whole business from the outset.

Your loved one will be on an increasing number of pills and potions as dementia advances, and they will also have been awash with them if Parkinsons was the illness which preceded it. It is essential to ensure that your loved one agrees to your being present at medical consultations, otherwise your life will become even more messy.

The next problem is that of who is responsible for prescribing and dispensing the medication. It could be the GP, the practice pharmacist, a specialist nurse, a consultant either in the hospital or the community mental health group, and so it goes on.

Then the word has to be passed on to the dispensing chemist, and if the medication is dispensed in weekly trays, be very aware of the fact that there may be a delay in shifting from one medication to another.

See my Parkinsons book for the full tale of woe that can unfold in such cases (pp. 40ff).

If you come up against intractable problems, especially when the magic phrase Patient Confidentiality is thrown into the mix, you should pass the buck to the specialist community nurse who looks after your loved one's case. That applies also in situations where the loved one has difficulty with medication or refuses to take it.

(j) Family history

This may seem a less urgent matter, but if you are in the beginning years of caring for a loved one with PD or dementia, one idea I heartily recommend is to encourage your loved one to put together a family history illustrated with images from the past.

It proved invaluable when Rusalka entered a care home, and we read through it, showing her the images of the family. It helped – or so it seemed – to reinforce her memories and imprint them on her.

The family history could then be saved on a USB and become a special personalised Christmas present for family members, especially the younger ones for whom our past is ancient history. We had countless family photographs to choose from and employ as illustrative material.

In the early days of her diagnosis, Rusalka was keen to undertake projects and we would spend time together working out what she wanted to achieve. These family histories, together with (in our case) pretty complicated family trees, formed one such project, and greatly helped to give her a sense of purpose and direction.

(k) Keeping a journal

Encourage your loved one to keep a journal recording daily events, feelings and concerns. She destroyed most of her entries as she became less well, but I came across these poignant words that Rusalka wrote in 2017:

> I prepared a timetable/schedule so that we could remember from one day to the next: shopping lists, appointment times, to even calling family and friends for a chat. I dislike going out as it is such a palaver using a hoist in the

> rear of the car. It is also so restricting. Takes me hours to get ready, when it was only minutes before my pain.

Those few sentences encapsulate so clearly how she declined over time, and how simple tasks could turn into huge challenges for her. The hoist was an electrically-operated device which enabled me to lower her motorised wheelchair in and out of the car, and it was very straightforward to use.

In her eyes, however, it constituted a serious obstacle to her mobility outside the house, and the last sentence of the extract underlines the odd way in which her insight varied so greatly. She was indeed painfully aware of the time it took her to cross a room, but she was unable to overcome her obsessive behaviour.

Chapter four – A dementia-friendly home

Before looking at the next item, here's a word of general advice when considering keeping your loved one safe in your home. Never go for just one solution to a problem. Two's company, and three is better still.

This is a significant issue which seems to have been almost totally ignored by the extensive literature surrounding dementia. If you cast an eye further along this chapter to the subject of user-friendly doors or personal alarms, you will see what I mean. There are any number of options to consider, and you should not make a final choice or choices until you have mulled them all over. Quite often, more than one solution should be put in place.

One further point to make is that you should also consider your own likely future needs and incorporate solutions for yourself as you go about improving the house for your loved one.

I am very glad that we were able to make changes round the house to ensure that it would be friendly to Rusalka both practically and from a dementia-friendly point of view. It was a five-year project and well worth it.

Do bear in mind the fact that, as more and more men and women live for longer with a range of disabilities, so an ever larger market place is growing for products of every shape and size, with tempting offers and special deals. Your big advantage, if you are planning well in advance, is that you do not have to rush into a decision.

Get as much advice as possible, from online sources and professional carers who visit many homes on a daily basis and can witness these products in operation.

The sections which follow are not in any particular order; in fact, I did at one point try and organise them but gave up trying. Not all of the sections refer to every situation, of course, so cherry pick your way through what follows.

A word of warning though: be very wary of telling yourself that you will surely not ever need a particular item. Think long and hard before discounting any individual suggestion of mine.

In writing this chapter I am very aware that I may not cover every eventuality, especially if your loved one has additional needs (hearing or sight problems, for example), and also that there are cost implications in just about every paragraph. Seek help and support if your finances are constrained. Your local authority social work department is the place to call for information. Check on the website for your council area.

(a) Flooring
We converted nearly all the ground floor rooms to wooden flooring, so that a wheelchair or rollator could move easily about. Laminate is a less expensive option. Do ensure that whoever is fitting such flooring does not create lumpy thresholds between one room and the next.

If at all possible, make the passage between one room and another entirely smooth. The smallest of thresholds can be bad news if your loved one is in a wheelchair or pushing a rollator or Zimmer frame. Believe me, we learned that the hard way.

Avoid rugs which can cause your loved one to slip and fall. Do ensure that there is space for a wheelchair or other equipment to move freely about the various rooms in the house.

(b) Grab handles
Next up are grab handles to help your loved one lift themselves upright, and do take account of the height they should be placed at. It is particularly important to have such handles in the shower or round a bath.

I found some manufacturers of grab handles – just google 'non-slip grab handles' – who incorporate rubber or similar rings on their products. Chrome throughout looks pretty, but you can easily slip if you have soapy hands, and that can be far from ideal.

(c) Local authority supplies

Your local authority or NHS Board have stocks of all kinds of supports, from bath seats and wheelchairs to commodes and devices to help your loved one out of bed. They can be loaned out to you on request. Our local authority helped us to purchase one of those fancy toilets which water spray the appropriate body parts after use, then dry them off with a hot air blast.

(d) Lifts and stair lifts

If your accommodation has two or more floors, you have to decide where you want your loved one to have access. In our case, we have one large upper floor room with an adjacent toilet, which we have used as a joint office.

Rusalka wanted access to this, not least because the cupboard space was groaning with handbags and shoes, and half the shelving accommodated her extensive collection of cookery books. It soon became apparent that climbing the stairs, even with additional handrails, was out of the question, so we explored the two options remaining: a personal lift and a stair lift.

We had two problems: the stairs were far too narrow to allow for a stair lift, not least because of a 180 degree turn near the top, and, secondly, there was not enough space for a lift which could accommodate a wheelchair.

So we opted for a lift plus an additional rollator or wheelchair for the upper floor. Installation caused quite an upheaval and is not exactly cheap. However, in our case it turned out to be a godsend, not least because of my own severely arthritic knee which ripened about the same time that Rusalka went into full-time care, meaning that the lift for me became a necessity.

If you live in accommodation with the bedrooms on the upper floor, you should consider converting one of the ground floor rooms into a bedroom, as a more cost-effective solution. You will need an adjacent toilet, too. Alternatively, you can obtain a portable commode in a wheelchair.

(e) Bath and shower

There should ideally be space within a shower area for a seat to accommodate your loved one. Standing for any length of time in a shower can be disorientating and tiring, especially if hair washing is involved.

As for a bath, this might seem an ideal opportunity for relaxation, but practicalities can soon get in the way. Baths are designed for able-bodied folk to clamber in and out of, and we acquired a walk-in bath, which unfortunately hardly ever gets used, as Rusalka went into full-time care soon after it was installed. I prefer showers.

(f) Commode

The chamber pot is a thing of the past, but the commode chair can be an essential piece of equipment for your loved one.

When is it most likely to be needed? Put simply, when your loved one 'needs to go' and the nearest loo is out of range. This can happen either during the day or at night, of course, and the requirement is most necessary when mobility is a serious issue.

At night, a commode by the bedside can be essential, because of the difficulties which can be experienced in clambering in and out of bed.

(g) User-friendly doors

Imagine yourself sitting in a wheelchair and trying to open one of the internal doors of your home. If it opens away from you, that's not too bad, but trying to pull it towards you is something of a nightmare, as the wheelchair keeps getting in the way and you cannot reach far enough.

So, what solutions did we come up with? The first involves thinking out of the box and considering which doors are actually necessary at all. Our cottage was built in the nineteenth century and a ground-floor extension was added with three bedrooms and a bathroom just before we purchased it.

The extension had a door fitted to the corridor which led to three bedrooms and a shower/bath/toilet. So the best solution was to remove it altogether or just wedge the door fully open. If you don't fancy a radical option like dispensing with the door, think next of ways of making the door easily useable by your loved one in a wheelchair.

The first thought which came to mind was to fit a roller ball catch to the door with a longish loop of material (a redundant curtain tieback) to allow her to reach forward and pull the door towards her. In the other direction, she could simply push the door open with the wheelchair.

I might as well mention collateral damage at this point. Wheelchair plus paintwork repeatedly meeting head on is not a good idea, so you may consider a metal panelling on the lower part of the door to reduce scuff marks and worse.

That is a reasonably inexpensive interim solution. Next up is the saloon door option, familiar to anyone who has watched a Western film, in which our hero pushes through the sculpted double doors with six-guns blazing.

I suggest that you explore using two doors rather than just one on double action hinges, for two reasons in particular. First, space. Two smaller doors opening in a relatively confined corridor, for example, take up less room than one large door. And the second point is that it is more difficult for your loved one to push against one large door than two little ones.

The next choice to consider is a sliding door. When I explored this possibility, I came up against two problems. The first was that, in those cases where a sliding door would work well, there was a radiator in the way, and we would have to factor in the cost of a heating engineer to shift it.

Problem number two is that some doors, notably those at the end of a corridor, don't have any wall on either side for the sliding door to move along.

However, if you do find that this is a possibility, do consider carefully which of the many variations on sliding doors is the best for you. I suggest one which is suspended on a sturdy metal rail. Ensure that the handle height is convenient for your loved one to reach easily.

The nuclear option is to go for an electrically operated door with a push button switch on either access point, plus a remote control for various functions, like automatic and permanently open.

I have a confession to make here. I went for this choice in the corridor leading to the main bedroom, and it was not a great success, to put it mildly. First, such doors do not exactly come free with the beer, to coin a phrase, and secondly, I did not anticipate how difficult it would be for a loved one with incipient dementia to cope with the various options for operating it.

So, the moral of all this is: think through all the options carefully before deciding which, if any, to use. Even consider as the first choice my earlier suggestion of either removing the door altogether or as a short-time solution, propping it open with a door stop to see how that works.

(h) Bedtime
The choice of bed is one item for which good forward planning can be extremely useful, particularly on the financial front.

Can I suggest that if you opt for an electrically adjustable double bed, you should be patient and wait for an end of season sale, as they can be seriously expensive and occasional discounts can be considerable, if you are prepared to hunt around for them.

Each side of the bed operates separately, and the main benefit is that the head can be raised or lowered to suit your individual requirements. The foot of the bed is also adjustable and this can be beneficial, too. I am not impressed by the vibrating options, though, as they just made my false teeth rattle, but other views are available.

Now for a word of warning, which had me baffled for quite some time. What happened was that after a while the remote controls on the bed went into a sulk and refused to operate.

I tried everything (or rather, as you will see in a moment, nearly everything) to persuade them to behave themselves. Changing the batteries did not work, neither did swapping the remotes from one side to the other.

Crawling underneath and checking out the wiring did not wave a magic wand, either, and I was beginning to think in terms of getting another bed at some considerable expense, when one of the remotes suddenly decided to play ball.

To cut a long story short, I discovered that Rusalka had emptied the pull-out drawer on her side of the bed so that she could check through the pillow cases, and the receiver box for the signals from the remote was now able to take orders from the remote control. The drawer-full of bedding was the guilty party: it had made it impossible for the receiver to respond to the remote.

Solution: move the receiver towards the edge of the bed until the remote control gets back on speaking terms with it.

As a footnote, we tried various other devices from the local NHS provider to adjust the height of the pillows, but none was particularly satisfactory, because they would tend to slide along the bed.

(i) Seating
If your budget permits, consider one of those chairs which tips forward to decant your loved one without them having to struggle upright, with the opposite function of being able to tip backwards as a kind of day bed.

Do ensure that the remote control is within easy reach of your loved one. Try placing a standard lamp next to the chair to improve lighting for reading or other activities, and then fix the remote to the side of the lamp. I used a small butcher's hook and a few lengths of insulating tape.

(j) Alexa and friends
One of the most rapidly developing technologies is voice recognition, and the ability of cheap equipment to obey commands delivered in ordinary speaking tones. Keep an eye open for further developments as they occur.

These devices are becoming pretty inexpensive, although you will require a wifi connection for them to function. The two main contenders are Alexa (who can be renamed, if you wish) and Google Assistant.

The great advantage of these systems is that they operate hands off, so making life easier for your loved one. They can perform all manner of tasks, including turning smart room lights on/off (and various colours, too), acting as a calculator, weather forecaster, radio station tuner, Audible book reader, music player, telephone, TV controller, front door bell answering, and more. The options grow by the day.

(k) Outside the building
If you have a garden, do think in terms of your future ability or otherwise to maintain it. We converted grassed lawns into gravelled areas, but do be aware that these can be difficult for some wheelchairs to struggle through.

We also installed a ramp with a side railing from the front door and a paved area next to where the car was parked. That proved essential when every step became a challenge for her, although I wondered if the expense was worth it when it was first put together. It was. Think long when you consider future needs.

(l) Wheelchairs and other equipment
This is a complicated subject, as they come in all shapes and sizes, powered and unpowered, so my best advice is to consider all the available options before deciding. My approach was to buy three, plus a rollator.

Please do note that the rollator comes in two flavours: three-wheeled and four-wheeled. We found the latter more useful, because it was more stable and the one we acquired had a seat which enabled Rusalka to pause for rest when she was out and about. Sudden tiredness is common with dementia.

Stools are also invaluable, including a raised step for helping her clamber in and out of bed. Also useful was a 'standing seat' to enable her to prepare food on worktops before it became too risky for her to wield a knife without endangering herself and those within swinging distance.

I have referred already to the usefulness of a stool in the shower, as prolonged standing is not beneficial and can lead to a slippery fall.

(m) Personal Alarms
I will be brief. This topic is covered in my first book, and is a clear example, in my view, of people leaping on one solution and believing that it will work in every circumstance.

It will function, provided that (a) your loved one doesn't lose the press button, (b) he or she remembers what it is for when she falls or has other problems needing urgent attention, (c) there isn't a power cut, and (d) if she is not at the far end of the house, which means that when the monitoring service asks her what the problem is, she is way too far out of range hear it and to reply.

My solution? I bought a couple of old-fashioned bulb horns as used by cyclists. They could be heard all over the building, even when the power was off.

(n) Helping hands
Discuss with your local authority the support you can get from carers who call into your home to check medication, assist with dressing and showering, and so forth. This is an invaluable service.

We also employed a cleaner and a gardener. Check out local charities for the kind of support they can offer.

Consult local authority and government websites. For example:

www.mygov.scot/care-equipment-adaptations

www.gov.uk/apply-home-equipment-for-disabled

www.gov.uk/apply-home-equipment-for-disabled – available for England and Wales residents only.

Now I turn to the most important part of the advance information you will need as your loved one's illness progresses.

Chapter five – Being prepared as a carer

One caveat to bear in mind is that, no matter how much factual information you acquire to help you cope with the person you are caring for, the emotional and mental issues which you will confront will still remain exactly the same. You may know 'as a fact' how to manage a particular set of circumstances, but that won't take away the pain and distress which is caused.

Also, do remember that the person you care for is not a collection of symptoms. A related point to make here is one that arises a lot in the literature about caring, and that is, that you should not bully or coerce your loved one. Try insofar as is possible to remember that they are people, not empty shells, and they need to be respected. More of that later in this chapter.

This can all be pretty challenging, especially when the loved one is particularly unkind in their responses to you, not least because all the manuals tell you: 'do not take it personally'. How else are you expected to react in such a personal situation? At best, you can mask your own feelings in that moment, but they will come to haunt you later.

What I have been struggling to put into words in the previous paragraphs is that, although it is vital for you as a carer to be prepared in advance for any challenging situations which will arise as you care for your loved one, that does not mean that you will be any less intensely aware and emotionally sensitive to those challenges.

On top of that, you may argue that I cannot possibly offer comprehensive help to you based on my experiences which are limited to just one person. Remember, I'm just an ordinary carer, an 'informal carer' at that, to use the common phrase which I find pretty insulting, and I cannot possibly be expected to cope with a hugely complex issue in which I have not had the benefit of any training, can I?

In reply, I'd say that is a counsel of despair, because it argues that no one can ever fully master any complex subject on the planet. It all depends on your mindset and how you approach such matters.

In addition, if I did throw the book at you, literally, containing all the facts and statistics ever compiled on the subject of dementia, you would require a huge yellow JCB with a very copious bucket to even lift the volumes of information you would have to try and absorb. The old proverbial phrase about not being able to see the wood for the trees comes to mind.

My approach to any subject is that no one can possibly be all-knowing about any one discipline, but that we can all manage to cope, given an appropriate approach. We may not have the detailed factual knowledge, but we can acquire the techniques which enable us to deal with new and difficult challenges.

Let me illustrate this with the corny old chestnut about the posh city-dwelling gentleman in his Rolls Royce tourer who has become lost in the countryside. He comes to a halt when he sees an old country bumpkin puffing a pipe and leaning against a five-barred gate.

'I say, fellow,' our posh driver calls out. 'Can you tell me how to get to the village of Much Piddlington?'

A pause, and several thoughtful puffs later there comes the reply, 'If oi was you, zur, oi wouldn't start from here.'

(Legend also has it that the exasperated motorist responds that surely the man should know better as he has lived there all his life, hasn't he? Came the reply: 'No, zur, I haven't. Not yet.')

The point I am labouring is that it is entirely wrong to start approaching the issues of interacting with the loved one with dementia by swallowing whole several books full of facts, or by chewing indigestible chunks of Google and assuming that you can become an expert that way. You should start with your loved one.

This is as good a point as any for me to get up on my high horse on the subject of carers who think they know it all. We don't. And do not delude yourselves that googling will somehow make you better informed than those who have spent a professional lifetime studying and working with people who have dementia.

Facts are just facts. If you want to become knowledgeable, you need this formula: facts + experience (lots of it) = knowledge, and there is no shortcut. I have seen relatives holding forth about how the loved one's medication is all wrong, causing their decline, until someone gently points out that they have got hold of the wrong end of the stick and are shaking it furiously and to no good purpose.

By all this, I do not mean that you should act deferentially towards the professionals, far from it. Do not hesitate to ask questions and wonder why things are as they are. But do remember the cautionary tale of the two Martian spaceships which land on planet earth and report back their findings. The first lands in Piccadilly Circus in London, the other in the middle of a blizzard at the south pole.

Neither, as you might guess, comes up with a rounded explanation of what life on earth is like. And one more point: do not fall into the trap of self-delusion. Dementia is a nasty disease which gets nastier. Sometimes it does not advance to the worst level, but do not become delusional: your loved one is far from being a special case being let down by the professionals. Quite the contrary: they are doing their level best against almost impossible odds.

One other point I must shoehorn in here, and that is the claim which I have heard time and again that the loved one is becoming 'institutionalised' in the care home. This is nowadays most unlikely to be the case. You should try to think in terms of the loved one shrinking in their cognitive capabilities, and that their supposed institutionalisation is simply a reflection of the way in which their disease is intensifying.

Let me turn again to that buzzword which is much used but not entirely well practised by the professionals: 'patient-centred medicine'. Your loved one isn't a bundle of symptoms needing to be identified and then fed the appropriate pills. He or she is first and foremost a person, a human being like the rest of us, who happens to have dementia.

If you set out from that point, however limited your technical knowledge, you will arrive more happily at that imaginary village of Much Piddlington. You can also be extremely helpful in watching out for the manifestation of problems at an early stage, such as cognitive changes, insomnia, or the signs of approaching delirium.

Remember too: the loved one does not necessarily feel your pain, nor even recognise the pain they may inadvertently cause you. Rusalka did not. The world folk with dementia inhabit is radically different from our own.

Chapter six – General advice in advance

The list I am going to present to you is in no particular order, except for the opening section on general advice, which you really should consult first. Do read through all the list items below and then move on to examine each in turn. You won't remember all of the information you will be presented with, but you will have enough at the back of your mind to know how to act when one of these issues arises, at which point do return to this book and re-read the appropriate section.

As you will know, dementia is an extremely varied many-headed monster, so I make no claim to being entirely comprehensive. That's beyond even the weightiest medical tome on the subject, and there's one more word of caution.

Do not take my words as gospel: remember the misguided advice of the 'experts' during the years of Covid-19: they exhorted us to 'follow the science'. The slight problem about that mantra is that there is no such thing as '*the* science'. There may be a general consensus, as there once was that the universe is in a steady state (now we should all accept the big bang theory of how we eventually all arrived on this planet).

Such patterns abound in the history of science and medicine, where one particular orthodoxy holds sway for years, to be replaced by another, and so on, and they have been repeated over the ages. Ask Galileo, way back in the seventeenth century, one of the most famous examples, when he got into trouble with the Inquisition over his heretical view that the earth might just be orbiting the sun, rather than the other way round.

Also there still is, lurking in dark corners of the health service, an inexplicable nostalgia for the bad old days of what I call medical medicine, the notion that 'for every ill, there's a pill', and that you shoot down the symptoms one at a time like ducks in a fairground show until a cure is achieved.

Now here comes the first set of pieces of help and support, which you should be aware of when dealing with your loved one.

(a) Don't take it personally.
This is an important but extremely challenging component of your interactions with a person with dementia. You loved one can be unintentionally cruel and hurtful, especially when there is a high level of paranoia present.

On days like that I can find myself being accused by Rusalka of all manner of crimes against humanity, including gallivanting with my mistress(es) or squandering all our money and bankrupting the family. Your loved one will not recognise or share the pain you feel when making those accusations, and in no time at all they will forget they have made them. You, unfortunately, will not.

As I have pointed out in the predecessor to this book, it's the carer who is closest to the loved one who gets it in the neck. That is just one of those facts of life for you to face, and you simply have to try and deal with it. There is no easy opt-out.

The harsh reality is that your loved one is no longer the same person as they were before the disease struck, and you have to accept them as they are, not as they once were or as you would wish they could be again. If their anger is especially directed at you, remember that, as the person closest to that loved you, you will inevitably be on the receiving end of most opprobrium.

Do also bear in mind that they will become more mentally frail as time goes by, and that even an unintentionally hurtful word or action on your part can be painful for them. Unfair, perhaps, but this isn't a matter in which fairness plays any role.

(b) Do not boss or order your loved one about.
Remember, people with dementia are not out of their minds entirely and just a bunch of cranky symptoms, as the old discredited medical model of the patient would have it. They are whole persons, in some respects diminished, so treat them with

respect and try and work within their ability to accept or agree to a course of action.

We all react inappropriately now and then, and that is just a result of our stress levels and exasperation at the inability of your loved one to behave as they did in the past. It's OK to make mistakes and put your foot in it. That is as good a way of learning from experience as there is.

One example will illustrate what I mean. When Rusalka was still back in our home with me, I purchased clocks which told the time, the day of the week, the date, and other information. After she went into full-time care, she indicated that she would like to have one of those clocks, so I dutifully obliged. Coming to visit her a couple of days later, I found the electronic face of the clock blank and the cable had gone walkabout.

Many husbands and wives have pet names for each other, some of which are seriously embarrassing, but the name which Rusalka acquired in this context was Tinkerbell. Not because she was fairylike, but as a result of her compulsive behaviour and determination to mess about with things.

Tinkerbell strikes again, I thought, counted up to ten and removed the clock. On the next visit, I produced a battery-powered clock, sourced on a well-known online selling site, and proudly deposited it on her side table.

Two days later, the clock lay on the table with a blank face, the rechargeable batteries had vanished and the press-button panel for setting the time, etc, damaged beyond repair. I actually got rather cross and told her so, which was exactly the wrong thing to do, and it distressed her. A lot. She could not get her head round the fact that she had done anything amiss.

Two days after that, I appeared with another all-singing clock and the care home handyman in tow. The clock had a screw-fastened top on the batteries and I asked for it to be affixed to the wall out of her reach. We were able to joke about the new arrangement and, fingers crossed, the saga of the clocks is over. Does anyone want to buy a battery-operated clock, broken and secondhand (pun intentional)?

Making an effort to learn from your mistakes and to try and find a way of non-confrontational interaction with your loved one takes time and patience, but the rewards can be considerable and beneficial to both of you in the long term.

Mental issues

(a) *Communication and distraction.*
Try and divert your loved one's attention away to some other topic if a problem with communication arises. This is particularly useful when they get stuck in a loop. How do you do that?

It requires a little mental agility on your part, and some practice, too. What you should do is rather like the misdirection which magicians exploit in order to enable them to perform their tricks.

Say, for example, your loved one accuses the nurse of stealing her sweets. Ask if she would like it if you brought her some chocolate on your next visit, or switch subjects altogether. Turn to a different topic, like what time the next meal is going to be served, or if she watched the news on her TV that day.

If you have to pause for thought before responding, remember what I learned when lecturing to students. A ten-second pause for thought on my part might seem an eternity, but for the students it's just a great opportunity for them to catch up on their note-taking. By then you should have got your thoughts together.

(b) *Short-term memory loss.*
I am reminded of the words of a nurse in the care home, whom I approached one day after leaving my wife in her room. I told her that Rusalka was distressed at my departure, and she replied that I shouldn't worry, she'd go into the room and invite my wife to visit the common room where some group activity was in

progress. Rusalka would then almost instantly switch into a more cheerful mode and my visit would vanish into the dark recesses of her mind.

This is an aspect of dementia which still catches me unawares. Only yesterday, as I write this, I arrived just after 1.30pm for a visit, and Rusalka complained that she had not yet had her lunchtime pills. So I toddled off in search of the staff, and after lots of toing and froing and much consulting of sheets of patient records, they determined that she had, in fact, taken her pills some time before.

I apologised profusely to the nurse charged with the distribution of medication and returned to Rusalka who, by that time, had entirely forgotten that she had claimed she had not been given her pills. So I wisely forgot it, too, and showed her photographs I had taken of the apple trees in the garden which were now in blossom, along with the cherry trees and the carpet of bluebells under the copper beeches.

(c) compulsive/repetitive behaviour
Two of my wife's actions under this heading might well strike a chord with you. I have already touched on her repetitive questioning about what time or day it is, so do acquire a clock which can help answer those questions.

Second up for my wife was another example of compulsive behaviour which manifested itself when she was still living at home and was able and keen to go out shopping, or when a dental or doctor's appointment was in the offing. If I told her that it was time to leave, it would often take her at least an hour to finish her make up, find a handbag and move from one room to another until she finally arrived at the front door.

The world record for her in this field was two hours. I also featured in the world nail-biting contest, waiting for her to emerge. She simply could not stop herself from earning her nickname of Tinkerbell with every object, large or small, that she chanced upon. Her travels across the house were increasingly blighted by what I called 'picking flowers along the way'.

That phrase goes back to an old German joke about the 'Bummelzug', literally a strolling local train, a very leisurely service whose journeyings were so casual that officialdom allegedly erected signs in the carriages warning that it was 'streng verboten', seriously forbidden, to pick flowers during the journey.

She would inch across a room, stopping at every object which interested her, and, believe me, there were many, and picking up some trifle examine it leisurely, and then replace it exactly where it was, leaving me silently fuming and gently trying to point out that if we take much longer it will be too late to go out at all.

The Institute of Advanced Motorists once had a watchword 'defensive driving', and that stance should be adopted with your loved one. It involves anticipating the faults of poor drivers and turning the other cheek, as it were, when most of us would be winding ourselves up into a state of road rage.

Our knee-jerk reaction might well be to respond in kind to bad driving, but taking defensive action can actually save lives. However, I do understand that it is pretty unsatisfactory that the bad driver will have learned nothing from the incident and will not 'go and sin no more'.

After much head-scratching, I could only find a couple of ways of coping with this behaviour: tell her a lot earlier that a trip out was in prospect and factor her involuntary delaying tactics into the process, and, secondly, helping her to have ready all the clothes, handbags, etc. for the trip out. When she could be persuaded to leave the bedroom, I'd take her by the hand and gently try and guide her past the many flowers lying by the wayside to which she was so addicted.

Another alternative was to try telling her that she was going out when I had already managed to manoeuvre her near the front door, but that often spectacularly misfired when she suddenly recalled that she had left some vital possession in the bedroom, at the far end of the house or that a visit to the toilet had urgently arisen.

The moral of all this is that prevention is better than cure and do aim to become a 'defensive carer'.

Such repetitive behaviour is very common, particularly asking what time it is, what day it is, and so on. If you just abruptly tell the person you're caring for what the time is, you have only resolved the problem for a short while, because the question will be asked again and again.

Try not to become exasperated if the question is posed repeatedly. Again, this is a reflection of the different world the person with dementia is living in. If you can, gently move the topic of conversation away, asking if it is time for tea, for example, what the weather was like the day before, and so on.

'Where am I?' 'And why am I here in this place?' That's a question which arises out of the blue occasionally, and it poses another difficult challenge. In Rusalka's case it's linked with the painful challenge: 'Why am I here at all and not at home with you?' Again, be tactful and be mindful of the mantra: Do not take this personally.

I hold her hands and look straight into her eyes and then I reply something along these lines: 'You are here because we all love you but we can't possibly look after you any more at home.' Then I swiftly move the subject away to something more congenial, before I turn into an emotional mess.

So let me sum up: it is important to be calm and unflustered by what appear to be deliberate 'delaying tactics'. You must respect the loved one's behaviour, which I know can be challenging when the dentist appointment looms and our country roads are peppered with slow-moving tractors and trailers which impede our progress, but you have to ensure that the timing somehow works out.

This is an important aspect of the 'patient-centred' approach, which can be very challenging for the carer, but do bear in mind that a domineering attitude might get your loved one more quickly into the passenger seat of the car on one occasion , but it will certainly not improve relationships over time, and it may well make the next similar situation more frustrating and a cause of ever greater disharmony.

It reminds me of the bad old days when I was a schoolboy and I asked for an explanation of a tricky problem from a teacher, who responded with a brusque 'Because I say so, boy.' A reflective pause followed by a helpful response demands a little more time, but it allows the pupil's perspective to be respected. However, there is no doubt that it calls for a radical shift of attitude on the part of the teacher. The same applies to other aspects of your role as carer, to which I now turn.

Chapter seven – Reacting as a carer

Here are some additional thoughts for you to consider in your dealings with your loved one.

(a) The value of 'active listening'.
If you have important information to pass on to your loved one, or if you just want to gain their undivided attention for a while, take their hands in yours, look directly at them, pause, and then speak slowly. Be prepared to repeat things, and do not rush through what you have to say. Remember their cognitive functioning operates at a slower rate that yours.

Rusalka, for example, had to give up driving, despite having long ago passed the Advanced Motorist driving test, because she simply could no longer process the incoming information and controls of the vehicle fast enough to be safe.

When discussing an important topic do remove distractions, by switching off the TV or radio, and drawing the curtains to prevent direct sunlight shining into their face. Ensure the room door is closed to reduce noise from outside.

You may well have to practise the same advice given to trainee teachers in the classroom: Say you are going to say it, say it, then say you've said it.

(b) Unequal relationship
I found many references in the literature about dementia to the notion of an 'unequal relationship', but it took me some time to become aware of just how unequal it is.

When your loved one was well, or just in the early stages of Parkinsons or Alzheimers, you were still able to interact with them as husbands and wives (or other relationships) do on an everyday basis. A great deal of informal negotiating takes place and decisions are arrived at together, unless, that is, the relationship is less than satisfactory in the first place.

When your loved one becomes less well, the balance of the relationship shifts almost imperceptibly at first, then more swiftly, at which point I came to recognise what the researchers meant by an unequal relationship. All the decision-making which was jointly arrived at now shifts into the hands of the carer.

(c) Slow down
Ensure that you proceed at the pace of your loved one, and don't impose your own on them. However, some days are better than others, and if your loved one is not communicating as well as usual, it is probably best to hold back on the verbal interactions, take their hands and just be physically present for them.

In teaching, I referred students to the curve of forgetting which I discovered is actually a serious scientific theory, baptised the Ebbinghaus curve of forgetting. The idea goes something like this: if you are told a fact, like 'the French for parrot is perroquet' and simply leave it at that, the bird flies away, so to speak, and is swiftly forgotten, unless you know how and when to intervene with a reinforcement.

My approach was that if you introduced new information, you should reinforce it the next day, then two days thereafter, then the beginning of the next week, and by then the curve flattens, and it should be permanently retained in the memory. Whether this works or not with dementia folk I'm far from sure, but it is worth trying on a shorter time scale.

My observation, for what it's worth, though, is that once short-term memory is impaired, there is no way of 'mending' it fully. Curiously, perhaps, long-term memories do remain intact for far longer, and you can exploit this when communicating with your loved one.

(d) When the sun goes down
Now that's an intriguing thought. What I'm referring to is a phenomenon which had me baffled when first I came across it, namely, what's known in the trade as 'sundowning'.

I came to notice not only that the illness did not progress on a smooth trajectory, but wobbled from one side to the other, if you see what I mean. She would have relatively good days and relatively bad days, both of which were as far as I could determine, not caused by any external factors.

Not only that, but I realised also that she had better and worse times during each individual day. In her case, the mornings could be particularly trying, but she would get better during the day and late afternoon was her best time. Then she would go downhill again.

This section is concerned with the state of the loved one during an individual day. And, to do so, we have to get a bit technical for a moment. Jargon alert coming up.

You may not have heard of circadian rhythm. It refers to the internal clock we possess which allows us to know roughly what time it is and helps manage our sense of time. It wakes you up in the morning, tells you when it is around lunchtime and sends you off to bed at night.

However, one of common features of dementia manifests itself when the circadian rhythm of the person with dementia fails to act properly. This has been baptised as 'sundowning', and a sundowner, apart from being a liquid refreshment taken at around sunset, is a person who suffers from this abnormality, which is most common in the more advanced stages of Alzheimer's or dementia.

Some times of the day are better than others for the person with dementia, and that is why I usually visit my wife in the early afternoon, as she has always been an owl rather than a lark, preferring the latter part of the day.

(e) Trust your own judgment
And, last but not least, don't be afraid to get things wrong. It is almost inevitable when interacting with a loved one that misunderstandings or minor differences between you will emerge

from time to time, and it is up to you to smooth over them and use your skills to divert attention away from them.

However, if things do go badly amiss, do not despair. Failure as a result of trying should not be regarded as a fault, but part of our constant learning processes as human beings. Here is an appropriate quote by Nelson Mandela: 'Do not judge me by my successes, judge me by how many times I fell down and got back up again.'

While I am in quoting mode, here's another on this topic from a quite different source, namely, Mae West: 'I never said it would be easy, I only said it would be worth it.' Our journey as carers is hard, and becomes ever more challenging as the months and years go by, but learning to be confident that you are doing your level best, even when matters get out of hand, is a vital part of your armoury.

Chapter eight – Foot in mouth

When interacting with your loved one, there are a number of stumbling blocks you will have to navigate around. These are all compounded by the cognitive deficit in your loved one, their slower pace of thinking, their sensitivity to negative reactions, and the fact that they are experiencing the world about them in a quite different way from the norm.

Much of what follows is concerned with what you should avoid, and is related to the notion of 'defensive driving' which I introduced earlier. Remember that it has two elements to it: on the positive side, it encourages you not to put your foot in it, but on the negative side, it can leave you frustrated that the strategy doesn't 'improve' the conduct of your loved one. That is a burden and you will just have to bite the bullet and bear it.

(a) Talking about the past

It seems uncontroversial to begin to chat about memories by saying something along these lines, 'Do you remember that holiday by the sea when a seagull stole all your sandwiches?', or 'Can you tell me what you had for lunch today?'

To tell the truth, this did not occur to me as a pitfall until I read about it in the literature. The reasoning behind the problem is that it imposes too much thought processing on the loved one, given that their recollection of recent and more distant past events can be very deficient.

As a result, posing a question which they find challenging to respond to causes anxiety and distress. This does not mean that there should be an embargo on such subjects, otherwise you might find yourself struggling to communicate at all with your loved one.

The advice is to think for a moment, and come up with an approach which it is easier for a response to be elicited other than 'I don't remember.' Here are my suggestions based on the two questions I noted at the beginning of this section.

First, the unfortunate incident with the seagull on holiday: 'I saw a couple of seagulls on the way in to see you, and that reminded me of the day when your sandwiches were stolen by a seagull. We were on holiday at the time and were staying in a caravan park.' then pause and see if that elicits a response.

And secondly, the food for that day's lunch: 'As I was passing the dining area just now, I think I smelled fish and chips. I know you love that dish. You used to make it regularly for the family, sometimes frying battered chicken breast instead of fish.'

Statements which might draw out a positive response are far less challenging than actually posing a question which forces the loved one to think hard and probably fail to come up with a reply, because their memory has let them down.

Do bear in mind, though, that memory is a weird and wonderful thing. A recent article in *The Sunday Times* colour supplement concerned a mother with dementia and her daughter. It was easier for the daughter to stay at home and not stimulate her, but one afternoon she took mother to the cinema to watch *West Side Story*. To her surprise, the older woman remembered the words to all the songs and joined in cheerfully.

From my own experience, Rusalka can remember quite specific events in the past, and she also retained some of the skills she had acquired in the past. Every day in *The Times* there is a 'word wheel', jumbled up letters to sort into a word, quite often of considerable obscurity. Before she fell ill, she could beat me at solving the puzzle nine times out of ten, and I still find that on a good day she can unscramble the letters almost as if nothing had happened to her.

This is not unlike the phenomenon of the 'savant', which in medical circles is used to describe someone with mental challenges, such as autism, who demonstrate remarkable skills in one particular area, such as mathematics, or drawing complex images from memory.

You should be aware of the fact that not all the abilities of your loved one fade at a uniform rate, and that you can be pleasantly surprised by patches of light in the growing darkness, so to speak.

(b) Right and wrong

This neatly follows on from the previous section, in that avoiding the problem is the best way of dealing with it. Quite often, your loved one will make a statement which is manifestly wrong. Out of the blue, Rusalka might say, 'There was an accident today and the ambulance came and took the lady to hospital.'

It's almost too tempting to respond with something like, 'Don't be ridiculous. You know very well there was no accident in the building.' Again, that response is hurtful and it challenges the loved one's perception of reality.

What is the best way of dealing with this issue? The answer is simple: Don't deal with it at all. Change the subject, divert their attention way to something quite different.

(c) Hallucinations

This is a similarly challenging area. Rusalka would often say something like, 'I saw my sister today. She's outside in the corridor now.'

Her sister lives a hundred miles away, caring full time for her husband, and unless she knows how to ask Scottie to beam her up and teleport her to the care home, there is no way that she can be around.

Once again, the worst reaction is to tell your loved one not to be ridiculous, as her sister is living many miles away with her husband. The right response is to divert the loved one's attention by making a general observation about the person referred to.

The same applies to auditory hallucinations.

One point to bear in mind: when Rusalka was only just beginning to slip into dementia, she was able to discuss these hallucinations, and their most striking aspect was how compellingly real they were to her, even though at that stage she was fully aware that they could not be true. So it is very important to deal sensitively with this aspect of dementia.

(d) I wonder how so and so is?
A rather touchy subject this, a variation on the previous section. Do be very sensitive in your response to questions about someone who has died, and who your loved one may believe is still alive and kicking. In Rusalka's case she would occasionally refer to her mother as if she was still among us.

Switch to a different topic to avoid unnecessary distress for your loved one. The question may be asked simply as a result of memory lapses or gaps in memory. Try to refer to the person at a later time and gently inform your loved one that they have passed away.

(e) Responding to paranoia
I am reminded of the old chestnut of the doctor who says, 'It's all right, Mr Jones. You are not paranoid. They *are* after you.' Reacting to paranoia in a loved one is particularly challenging, especially when you are the object of the paranoia.

This phenomenon can be at its most severe during and after a psychotic episode, and often takes the form of accusing you of being unfaithful, chasing after other potential partners and generally living a life of unrestrained debauchery.

This is the point where I really must repeat the mantra I've used more than once in this book: 'Do not take it personally.'

Chapter nine – Coping with dementia

What follows are more items which play an important role in the loved one's life but can easily get overlooked. They play a key role whether the loved one is at home or in a home.

Simple interventions in looking after your loved one as a whole human being can be very rewarding, and making an effort to anticipate the loved one's needs can help to keep things running as smoothly as they can. One such example from dealing with my own parents sticks very painfully in my mind. Many years ago, we travelled down from Scotland to visit my father, who was recovering from a serious operation in the ICU of his local hospital.

At first, the situation appeared to be pretty bleak and upsetting for all concerned, as he appeared disorientated and unaware of who we were. Also, he was incoherent and distraught, until I asked the nurse where his teeth and spectacles were. They were duly reinstated, and he was instantly transformed.

(a) What's the time? What day is it?
Your loved one will often ask you those questions, and sometimes repeatedly so. The practical response is to try and anticipate this with the help of one of those so-called 'dementia clocks'. I make no apologies for repeating myself here.

One further point: these clocks are evolving and getting better all the time: the one I most recently purchased had the option of a split colour display, with the time displayed as a digital readout on the right, and on the left as an old-fashioned analogue clock face. That could be easier for the person to understand, as that is the dominant form of time display and one which continues to be the default means of communicating the time.

Some of these clocks also offer the option of displaying photos via a USB stick, an option you can use with your loved one as a talking point for reminiscing.

(b) Loss of balance

This is not one of those issues in which you can simply state that there is one simple cause which can be removed to eradicate the problem.

Having hacked my way through piles of learned information on the subject, my instant facetious response is to place copies of the PDF document files I have slogged my way through at strategic points on the floor of our home so that they break Rusalka's fall.

In other words, you can take preventative measures by the bucket load but they won't stop your loved one from suffering a fall every now and then. I can only offer my own experience and hope that it informs your decision-making.

My best guess is that there is no single cause of falling, as the phenomenon is a symptom of something else which drives it. That 'something else' can be one of a whole range of causes, and they cannnot necessarily be traced back to dementia. It might simply be a case of trying to bite off more than you can chew, and that could be explained in terms of getting old rather than having dementia.

From my own observations, a fall most frequently occurs when your loved one's perception of a situation differs from the reality. Let me translate that into English. She reaches out for the arm of a chair for support, not realising that it is out of her grasp, she falls, and that appears to be caused by a difference between her perception of the reality of a situation and her actual inability to manage it.

What used to happen next was that Rusalka would become shocked, hysterical even, and the only way to manage that situation was to comfort her and allow the waves of unpleasant emotions she was experiencing to wash over her. In moments like that, I tell her that she shouldn't demand that I fetch the Air Ambulance for her, even though the helicopter is based just a few miles down the road from where we live.

You will find yourself accused of failing to act appropriately and of trying to make light of a genuine emergency, but that it just one more of the joys of being a carer. Unfortunately, she would relay that incorrect perception to other family members who would blame me for the fall in the first place and my uncaring response.

So, in my limited experience, falls will happen even though you could pad the entire house with cotton wool, and there is no way they can be prevented.

Having said all that, medication might be a contributory factor, and it is worth mentioning the fact to the doctor at your next visit if the falling becomes too frequent.

(c) Wandering

One of the commonest and most frightening tendencies of a person with dementia is the impulse to go walkabout without warning and often beyond the safe confines of the house or garden.

In the case of my wife, she fortunately restrained her wandering to the house and immediate garden, but it was still very concerning to see her comfortably sitting in her reclining chair at one moment and then the next to find she had vanished out of sight.

This can be extremely worrying for the carer and can also be distressing for the person you are caring for, but for quite different reasons. Once again, like falling, this is a situation where the loved one is over-reaching themselves, as the wanderer soon faces two dilemmas: Where am I; and How do I get back to where I was?'

Have a badge round her neck with name address and phone number is a sensible idea, if they will be prepared to accept it, that is. Particularly if the loved one isn't, as one might put it coyly, appropriately dressed for an outing into the locality, the sensible approach is prevention insofar as it is possible. Lock the front door, use the GPS function on their phone, if they have it with them, and hope for the best.

(d) Unwillingness to take medication
Use patience and persuasion. But if that does not work, try finding out if the medication can be administered in another form, liquid, for example. Also, if the medication is suitable for crushing, sprinkle the bits over a soup or sauce and let them take it that way. If the medication is suitable, that is.

Another important point for the carer to bear in mind: if changes in the medication are implemented, be on the lookout for new symptoms in your loved one. If any arise, contact your doctor in the first instance for advice on what action to take.

(e) Disturbed sleep patterns
This is a tricky one, as sleeping during the day for increasingly long periods of time can cause less rest at night. And the thought of Tinkerbell getting it into her head that she wants to boil a cup of tea and make some toast had me leaping protectively out from under the duvet and into the kitchen.

Your doctor and nursing staff should be made aware of the issue, and they should be able to assist in at least making the situation tolerable.

(f) Cognitive issues
The golden rules are: Be patient and do not get angry or show frustration at your loved one's responses. Don't make them self-conscious about their deficiencies in cognition. Also remember the golden rule: Don't take it personally. (Have I mentioned that already?) In other words, do not react in a hasty and self-protective way.

The person with dementia can view the world quite differently from most people, and you must bear that in mind.

(g) The five senses
It's almost inevitable that the senses will be negatively impacted by dementia. Again, this is something which affects people very

differently, and what follows is a mix of my experience with Rusalka and hoovering information from the internet.

Do be aware of the fact that as we become older, all our senses deteriorate, as do our means of processing what the senses are telling us. Having dementia amplifies and accelerates such changes.

Smell
This sense is not readily lost but olfactory hallucinations can be a very troubling phenomenon. My wife has often been plagued by the smell of burning, almost to the point of calling the fire brigade.

Smell can also be affected in a similar way to the impact on victims of Covid-19, where it can become almost completely wiped out. As smell and taste go hand in hand, so to speak, it's not surprising that it can then be one of the causes of eating problems for the loved one.

Hearing
If you have tried recording an interview in a relatively noisy environment, you will be surprised at how much of the unwanted ambient sound intrudes upon your recording. The reason for this is that our minds can cancel out many sounds when focussing on a particular voice or voices, whereas the dumb machinery just retains everything within its audio range.

There is evidence that this kind of indiscriminate audio intrusion is often to be found amongst people living with dementia, and loud noises can be particularly disturbing for them. Also, you may find that your sufferer's voice becomes quieter and quieter, and when they are asked to speak up, they protest that they are speaking at normal volume.

Hearing loss can cause isolation for the loved one. If you see signs of this occurring, take steps to arrange a hearing test; and also ask for a nurse to clear wax out, as this tends to accumulate in dementia.

Hearing aids can be very beneficial, but like all equipment they present problems of understanding and operation for the loved on. They can also so easily become lost, and do let me know if anyone has managed change a hearing aid battery without causing it to roll under the nearest sofa and disappear.

Vision
This can be very problematic, but I have not personally encountered distortions of vision in my wife. She has suffered from visual hallucinations, but that is a different issue from eyesight deterioration.

Rusalka has been particularly keen to point out patterns in, say, wallpaper or carpets, creating shapes (people and animals) where I could not perceive any. I did not give it a second thought until I read somewhere that this could be a sign of Alzheimer's or dementia.

At the time I was completely unaware of the fact that this skill was in fact a warning sign of future deterioration. It is common generally amongst those with dementia to over-interpret what their eyes are telling them, in other words, this is an information processing issue which requires sensitive handling.

Ensure that the loved one has spectacles to suit their condition, with back-ups in case of loss or damage. Rusalka would purchase additional reading glasses at knockdown prices from local shops.

Touch
Do continue to hug and touch your loved one, but try not to upset them in the process. Respond rather than taking the initiative. the loved one needs to feel loved, wanted and respected.

Taste
Reduction in tasting ability can cause the loved one to change their food likes and dislikes.

Summary

There is a related but different matter which has an impact on all the senses, and that is the reduced ability of the loved one to process incoming information, the Sunday name for which is cognitive impairment, which can also cause considerable problems. You should be aware of this and adjust your interaction with the loved one accordingly.

Like all medical conditions, dementia is a complicated beast and deterioration in one or more of the sense could well be a sign of an underlying problem, such as delirium or infection, so do keep the medics and care staff informed.

(h) Colours and their problems

The jury appears to be still out on the importance of colour and light for dementia patients. However, I have managed to distil a couple of general points. Blue is regarded as restful and blue food plates offer a clear colour contrast to food.

Red also offers a positive choice for food plates, but it is more of an attention-grabbing colour than blue. Green, by contrast, is very restful and is a good choice for decorating walls.

Pink apparently reduces aggression and that could also be useful for wall decoration. Black is contentious, as it can cause the loved one to see it as a dark hole in the ground, so black carpets are out.

Advice abounds, such as painting the doors of rooms contrasting colours (as well as putting an image and name plate to indicate their use), but this is an area which in general appears to me to be work in progress.

(i4) Don't contradict

Here I am at risk of repeating myself, but the following advice also applies in this context. The loved one will almost certainly say things which are plainly wrong. For example, if they state incorrectly that the staff have failed to give them the right medication, or that our pet dog's name was Judy, when we don't have a dog, you must constantly bear in mind the uncomfortable fact that their 'reality' is both diminished and in a different shape from that of 'normal' folk.

Challenging such assertions can do far more harm than good, and you should swiftly change the subject and move on. The advantage of short term memory loss (if you can describe it as such) is that your loved one will very rapidly forget what has just been said and will move on to something else.

(j) The incomplete sentence
Very frequently, your loved one will be talking away and then suddenly stop in the middle of a sentence. In Rusalka's case as I write, she is most often still conscious of the fact that she has forgotten a particular word or phrase, and invites me to complete her words.

In such cases, the most supportive approach is, I believe, to offer her three or four alternative words or phrases so that she can light upon the one most suited to her requirements. Here's an example: if she is talking about her clothing and is wanting to ask about a particular garment, run though a list of options, like dress, skirt, top, stockings, bra, and so on.

Either that, or I simply change the subject altogether. This is yet one more tricky issue, especially when the loved one is aware of the problem and looks to you for a solution.

Rusalka likes to have a notebook in which she records the events of the day, plus information she needs to have on paper. This is an invaluable way of helping her orientate herself. I referred at the beginning of Chapter two to the family histories she put together, which I am now compiling with her help into an electronic record of the family as a Christmas present later this year.

Store a number of photographs from the past on your mobile phone, if you have one, and show them to her to see if she recalls when they were taken, who was present, and so on.

(k) urinary or double incontinence

This is a distressing issue and one which needs careful management. I have only had to deal with the former, and I have found the best approach is to be very matter-of-fact in both helping her to keep her well supplied with disposable underwear, and also in mopping up after an unexpected spill on the floor.

That's another reason why wooden floors or similar are preferable to carpets.

It can sometimes be caused by the loved one simply forgetting to replace incontinence pads after a previous toilet visit, so I always perform a sensitive check to ensure that she has, and, if not, to repair the damage, so to speak, with as little fuss as possible.

I may be wandering into territory way above my pay grade here, but it is worth considering the kind of disposable underwear to purchase. If your loved one is in a care home, you may well find that they provide pads but not full pull-on protective wear.

If you can budget for it, do consider providing such wear, as it offers a tighter seal and does not require additional underwear to hold it in place, thus avoiding little golden puddles which can occur without warning.

Chapter ten – Coping with dementia (continued)

I have made a break at this fairly arbitrary point, because otherwise you might become overwhelmed by the information being thrown at you. The following items do also reflect a shift in emphasis, though.

(a) Problems with food

An agency carer once said accusingly to me: 'Rusalka isn't eating her dinner.' Not a well-trained person obviously, because the answer is that Rusalka wasn't being naughty or uncooperative. She could be (as I bit by bit worked out for myself):

> Forgetful and thinking she has already eaten it;
>
> Having difficulty swallowing the food and needs to see the speech therapist again;
>
> Has lost her sense of taste/smell and has therefore reduced appetite;
>
> Her perception of the food on the plate is distorted;
>
> Needs reminding of which implements to use for cutting and eating food;
>
> The food is too hot or cold;
>
> Losing a sense of taste. I can sympathise with that one, having suffered from it myself during and after a bout of Omicron;
>
> The colour/shape of the plate could be confusing to her;
>
> Confused with the cutlery – giving her too much choice, perhaps. Using a spoon as a knife, for example, and cutting at a strange angle. Not getting enough food in the mouth and simply giving up;
>
> Needs help in cutting the food up;
>
> If eating alone, she should be invited to join other residents at mealtimes so that she can be encouraged to follow their example;
>
> Simple dislike of a particular food. Even people with dementia remember their culinary likes and dislikes;

Food too difficult to eat. Manual dexterity, or the lack of it causes her to push food off the plate instead of into the mouth.

Difficulties swallowing followed by vomiting. If the issue is reflux, consult a specialist nurse or doctor.

The list goes on and on. Use gentle questioning to try and determine the actual cause(s).

(b) Retail issues

What could be easier than taking your loved one out shopping? Actually, it can be fraught with issues of all kinds which raise some fascinating general points about the care of people with dementia in such settings. Using the precautionary principle, don't take your loved one out at all if there is a chance of problems arising because they are having a bad day.

Rusalka caused quite a lot of problems when she went shopping. Her favourite target was the charity shops, and she would push her rollator round loading it up with shoes, handbags and clothes, none of which she really wanted. It became well nigh impossible to persuade her to leave the shop, and that caused a lot of issues for others present. She now rarely goes out from the care home.

I came to these conclusions: (1) It wasn't her 'fault'. She had become locked in a loop, so to speak, and it was a real tussle to persuade her out of it. (2) Shop staff are not trained to deal with dementia or other disabled persons and that should be a priority, difficult to enforce when most of the assistance in charity shops are volunteers. (3) Shops are not designed to be dementia friendly, and that would be a challenging balancing act for the retailer.

Do also be aware of the fact that the person with dementia can accidentally leave the shop without paying, but still thinking they have done so. That can cause real problems, particularly if staff become officious.

(c) Psychosis (delirium or UTI related)
Delirium is a serious medical emergency, often caused by a UTI (urinary tract infection). It needs swift intervention, when medication may be offered to get rid of the UTI, or the loved one may even have to be admitted to hospital.

When the psychosis arises suddenly, UTI is the suspect of choice and it can usually be sorted with an appropriate antibiotic.

The second type is easier to recognise but no easier to treat. What happens over time is that the loved one's behaviour becomes more and more unusual until some trigger point sets off a full-blown psychosis.

(d) The need to go into a care home
Here are the main reasons, but for me the most important is the first:

> (1) The carer can no longer cope with an overwhelmingly demanding and unmanageable situation.

> (2) The safety of the loved one is at risk, particularly related to the tendency of many folk to go wandering.

> (3) There is a loss of bowel control, especially when the person cared for doesn't deal with it or recognise it as a problem.

I must stress one point here: if you have not been in the situation I have regarding extrremes of coping, do not rush to judgment. against me I was forewarned about this when my mother, who was caring for my father with dementia and bowel issues, phoned me one morning and said: 'I just can't cope any more.'

What the straw was that broke the proverbial camel's back in this case, none of us can tell, but believe me, it will happen. And it will not be your fault. All credit to you for having come further along this road than you would ever have believed possible, especially those who criticise you.

Chapter eleven – Visiting your loved one

This is an area which is least regarded and keenly important from the carer's point of view. For those not immediately involved – and I include the team of professionals around your loved one in this – it's like the final curtain of a play has fallen and the rest is incidental.

Now you can rise up from your seat in the auditorium, discard the programme, drive home and start anew. Oh, really? That is a travesty of what actually happens, and it can cause more grief to the carer than anything that has gone before. Trust me.

One of the surprising contradictions which hit me was the difficulty I experienced in coping with visiting Rusalka. Surely, you would argue, it is easier for you now. All you need to do is leap into the SUV, zoom off to the care home, spend an hour or so examining the wallpaper and come back refreshed and consoled that she is being looked after properly now.

Let me try and break this issue down into its main component parts:

      (1) You cannot cope with visits;
      (2) You cannot cope with the symptoms you observe;
      (3) You cannot manage yourself while you are away from your partner etc.;
      (4) Is this a one-off bad day?
      (5) Is this a situation where you no longer feel able to manage as an absentee carer at all?

I said to the manager of my wife's care home one day, 'I hesitate to put this feeling into words, but there are times when I ask myself what I am doing here.'

Her reply shocked and surprised me. 'Don't be concerned. It is a common source of worry. You are the second carer today to ask exactly that question and feel the same amount of guilt.'

The temptation to stay too long can be strong, but it should be resisted. Give your loved one the space to be alone or in the company of fellow residents, to be themselves and become settled.

Of course, you can say 'yes' to more than one of the above, which makes your situation even more complicated. Let me deal with these problems one at a time, if I can.

There are a lot of different issues all bundled up inside the main problem. Some are more easy to cope with than others, so let s look at what is involved.

First, you may find that the visit drags on interminably. One solution is to cut back on the amount of time you spend. There is no fixed ideal time per visit – it all depends on you and the person with dementia. The same applies to the frequency of visits.

A second solution is to vary the amount of time according to the state of mind of the resident. If he or she is rambling incoherently and not really acknowledging your presence, pick a moment to say that you have to go now, because you have other stuff to deal with.

Also, vary the content of your visit. What do I mean by this? Let me give an example from my years of lecturing to students. When I first started off, I would charge on through the hour from beginning to end, scarcely pausing for breath. However, I soon realised that two key elements of a really successful teaching experience were missing: change of pace and interacting.

In my lecturing days, during a session, halfway through I would learn to pause for a moment, come forward from behind the lectern to sit on a desk and present an off-the-cuff summary of the material I had covered thus far.

The other alternative, interacting, demands more confidence, gained by experience over the years. If I saw a student puzzled at something I have said, for example, I would ask them directly if I can help with anything from the spelling of a name to a complex theoretical proposition I had thrown at them.

Of course, the two can be mixed together, and a similar approach may well help to ease your time with the resident. One trick of the trade I would use, if the conversation has begun to pall, is to dip into a bag of goodies I had brought with me and present her with another one, like the monthly puzzle book I subscribe to her on her behalf, or an item of clothing or jewellery. They can be the trigger point for a renewed interaction.

Of course, if you bring with you a friend or relative this can allow the burden to be shared out, so to speak, but the downside to this comes if the attitude of your fellow visitor is less tolerant and patient than you have become. My view, for what it's worth, is that the resident appreciates full attention from a single visitor on whom they can concentrate and react to in an uninterrupted manner.

If you find the whole business still too challenging, seek help. This is a hit-and-miss situation, and one of the key reasons why I wrote this book. However, I was lucky to find that Alzheimer's Scotland5 had a local scheme running to allow for weekly phone calls from a counsellor to provide support and encouragement, which proved invaluable to me.

Do not expect to find that placing your loved one into a care or nursing home will make life easier. The exact opposite is likely to happen, as you will see now in Part three coming up. Take particular note of the chapter on anticipatory grief.

Part three – Caring for the carer

Chapter twelve – Who needs care?

Now here's an interesting question. When you are caring for a loved-one with dementia, who is it that needs love, constant attention, encouragement and support, in other words, who is the most important person in your life?

Your loved one, obviously. Wrong. The most important person is You. Now, at first sight that sounds strange, or even spookily pseudo-psychological. However, it does make good sense if you think about it. If you can't love yourself and take care of yourself, you are in no position to look after others.

Carers are notoriously bad at looking after themselves. They are sometimes stressed to the eyeballs (to use a non-medical term) and that doesn't just make them tired, it exposes them to all kinds of medical issues and illnesses. And if you are bedridden with anything from the flu to the plague, you aren't much use to your loved one. All that sets off a chain reaction the outcome of which is unpredictable.

You must also be conscious of the need to deal appropriately with your loved one. If they are causing you any concern, Do Something. Start by googling, then if necessary call the doctor. Much of the literature encourages you to go to support groups, and do so if they work for you. My flesh crawls at the very thought, but maybe I'm a complete outlier in this respect.

It is also vital to find ways of boosting your own morale. Even a half hour or so of respite will help you recharge the proverbial batteries, and give you the strength to carry on. If your loved one is annoying or upsetting you, which will happen with ever greater frequency as time goes by, remember, as I may have stressed elsewhere: Do. Not. Take. It. Personally.

It's the wretched disease talking, not your loved one. As I have stressed elsewhere, do not be either an optimist or a pessimist. Be a realist. Recognise that things will, with vastly varying rates of change, become worse, but remember also that there will be good days as well as the bad days.

You must also recognise that your relationship with the loved one will never be as it was before the illness struck. There is a lot of talk in the text books about happy marriages being a good foundation for the caring role as it develops. Nonsense.

Nothing can be a good foundation o prepare you for what is to come: the better the relationship, the harder it will be to come to terms with the new normal (to coin a phrase). And that is just one of the many issues that you have to deal with. The only consolation is that you will for most of the time be too busy caring to have time to brood and ponder.

In my own case, a family member is constantly leaping upon every positive aspect of the loved one's behaviour as proof positive that she is improving or at the very least plateauing at her current level. As a result, the loved one ends up being treated inappropriately and it all ends in tears, with the family member blaming everyone except himself.

Chapter thirteen – Educating carers

I have asked in many quarters and read extensively in this area: Is there support for carers? (I was a full-time 'informal' carer for my wife for over a decade.) Of course there is, comes the answer. Financial support is available, as is local authority support for staff to visit our home and help my wife with functions like showering and dressing; and carers may have respite and telephone/personal visiting, offering a shoulder to cry on.

But my main question, particularly significant now that her dementia is becoming more pronounced, is this: What formal organised support is there for offering *training* to all carers in how to interact with their partner or relative who has dementia when issues arise? I should have posed this question years ago, but I was too tired, emotionally drained, too busy being a carer and was having to make things up as I went along. I learned a lot the hard way, but I do not know if it is all appropriate or positively helpful to her.

Now that she is in a home, the problem becomes more acute. It is clear that she is deteriorating in many ways, but I have no expertise in how to interact with her on my regular visits. I understand that nursing and care staff can have such training, but we as carers are seriously being left out of the loop. My task is done, the feeling is, and I and others are 'just' visitors. Leave it to the professionals and don't trouble yourself (or us).

I would like to see all carers formally offered the chance to be fully aware of the skills required to manage these and a host of other situations where it is not easy to understand and react appropriately to the issues which the person with dementia is struggling. (Maybe, perish the thought, even being allowed to sit in on part of the training given to professionals.) It can also assist them to come to terms with a situation which is perhaps even more painful and intense than when physically caring for the partner, etc. It has been appropriately described in the literature as 'anticipatory grief', and it must be addressed.

Maybe it's because no one thought to ask, only an elderly nuisance like me. I really would like to be able to make a positive contribution towards improving this situation, and writing is the only thing I have the energy and skills left in my creaky old age.

The problem with the carer is that their role is not regarded as a medical condition, and that is certainly correct. However, I would regard it as a potential pre-condition to significant mental health issues.

Chapter fourteen – Facing 'anticipatory grief'

'Anticipatory grief', that mess of emotions which overwhelm you when your loved one goes into full-time care, is a complex and challenging phenomenon that can feel bewildering, intensely painful, numbing and overwhelming. And largely ignored by others, professionals included.

I am going to attempt to tease apart the tangle of emotions it embodies, most of all because it is important for you to know your enemy, so to speak. That is the first step towards overcoming it.

In its early stages, you hardly have the time to come to terms with it and recognise it for what it has become. As in any critical life situation – a death in the family, serious illness, a bad car crash – you are so caught up in the practicalities of this life-altering crisis that you fail to notice what is going on beneath the surface.

For a while, those practicalities take over. You may have to choose between more than one care/nursing home, there are financial arrangements to be made, small details like clothing, hair dryer, brush and comb, bottles of shampoo, toothpaste and the rest to be organised, dates and times decided upon, medication issues and a whole lot more to be sorted out and dealt with.

And then, all of a sudden, everything goes quiet. Your loved one has moved away, the fuss and bother has died down, and a routine of visits is settled upon. That's when you come to realise that your life has altered irrevocably and that you are being left more or less to your own devices in coping with this new and frightening situation.

You are now facing an uncertain future, and it may only gradually dawn upon you that you have a serious mountain to climb in coming to terms with all that has happened; or, as in my case, it can occur quite suddenly and without any warning.

I had returned one day from visiting Rusalka, a pretty challenging experience because she was going through a phrase of bewilderment and disorientation at her sudden change of accommodation and environment, and as the front door closed behind me, I instantly became painfully aware in that moment of the silence in the house.

The familiar little noises were still there, but they seemed to echo hollowly in the empty space – the hiccough of our cuckoo clock, the thunking and whirring of the central heating, even the drone of a neighbour's lawnmower, all of them reminded me that a familiar and precious collection of sounds was now missing. Rusalka's voice was no longer to be heard, the rumble of her rollator across the wooden floor, the sights and smells of a lifetime together, all vanished.

Do not think for a moment that this was purely an awakening to self-pity, although there was more than a hint of that in the equation. It was a recognition that two key aspects of my whole existence had been brutally and irrevocably torn away from me: my role as carer, and my relationship with my wife of so many years.

Those elements had been so central to my own life, and to have both swept aside so abruptly and cruelly, without any kind of preparation or foreknowledge, compounds the felony almost beyond endurance. The loved one in her new home has now become the focus of attention, and that is right and proper, but the carer is left high and dry to fend for themselves.

Let me be blunt. It is as if you have been sidelined, that you have been relegated into playing only a bit part in this real life drama. Your role is over now, and you can sit back and watch the world go by, or return to your former pleasures in life. But you can't.

This 'anticipatory grief' is almost worse than experiencing the actual death of a loved one, as the pain of bereavement continues without the sense of closure which 'normal' grief eventually brings. It's like a Greek tragedy without the catharsis – the purging of the emotions – which is one of its central objectives. The unpleasant emotions simply go on and on.

So, if there is no Good Samaritan to raise you up from the roadside and tend to your wounds, what do you do? What's the plan? How can you emerge from this darkness whilst the cause of it all – your loved one's removal from your care and your life – lingers on and the situation cannot be reversed or improved.

Everyone's circumstances are, of course, different. You may have a large circle of support, of family members and friends, to comfort you and ensure that a regular supply of frozen home cooked meals appears at your door. They can come round to the house, make the appropriate consoling noises, stay a while and then depart, probably relieved that the visit is over and they do not care to dally any longer in the presence of your emotional maelstrom.

But in nearly every case, none of those kind and caring folk has been through an experience remotely like yours, and you may well feel, as I did (and do), that this is a uniquely solitary kind of suffering which is yours and yours alone, one that cannot be fully or even partially shared with anyone else.

You feel that the very mention of your inner troubles would be met with an accusation of selfishness. After all, your loved one is being looked after for you and you are now as free as a bird. Don't grumble and look on the dark side, just 'pull yourself together' and enjoy your new-won liberty.

But where in all of this is there any proper support for the carer? Left alone, as you and I have been, there are many dangers that lie ahead to our own mental and physical health, and surely on a purely practical cost benefit analysis, prevention is better than cure. A spoonful of support at this key time from the professionals is so much better than a ton of aftercare when everything has gone really pear-shaped further down the line.

Consider the numbness you can experience: it's an odd kind of refuge from bad and excoriating thoughts and emotions, and although you recognise it as a not particularly positive place to be, it is a pretty dangerous No Man's Land to find yourself in. There is no one out there to share this hugely tangled web of emotions swirling within you. All you can do, it seems, is to sweep those feelings under the carpet and pretend they no longer exist.

Those who know about such matters claim that there are five or seven stages to grief. First, the shock and denial, then an overwhelming pain and guilt, like the survivor's guilt which confronts serving soldiers on the battlefield when their mate lies bleeding and they are physically unscarred. Next in turn come anger and depression, and in time, the beginnings of an upturn away from the anguish and despair.

The trouble is, in the case of anticipatory grief, instead of those stages coming sequentially, they all pile in together simultaneously as you confront the 'non-death' of your loved one. And that makes it all the more challenging for you to find a signpost to direct you away from the intensity of that potentially lethal cocktail of emotions.

Throw into the mix a sense of lacking direction and purpose, which is another common reaction to your changed situation, which drains away all those meaningful activities of the past and bleakly confronts you with the question: if she or he is no longer by your side, what is the point of having objectives? If there is no one to share them with, there is seemingly no rhyme or reason in aiming at a goal if you cannot turn to your loved one and share the experience together.

Hard though it may be, each of us has to map out our own path out of what John Buchan in his famous allegory *The Pilgrim's Progress*, called 'The Slough of Despond'. He was describing the supreme challenges confronting faith which the world can throw at you, and his narrative penned way back in the seventeenth century echoes down the ages to us in our modern mire of despondency.

I have found some consolation in tapping these words out on to the computer screen and hoping that they will not simply give you pause for thought, but also some way of scrambling out of all this mess, a renewed sense of purpose, although at my age of eighty-one, I wonder how long-term my objective could realistically be.

I hope you find your own path. It will not be easy, far from it, and as for the grief, it cannot be simply chased away. It will, we hope, fade gradually as the weeks, months or even years go past. Even then, there exists the daunting prospect of your loved one actually passing away.

When that occurs, you may well have already done all your grieving, and what remains is a deep well of sorrow mingled with some gratitude that you at least experienced good years way back in the past. Surely we cannot twice experience the intensity of that 'anticipatory grief'.

I hope that some at least of the advice and information I have offered will be of use and support for you in your continuing journey with your loved one. I wish you well.

Endpiece

Sources

In my previous book, I avoided a bibliography, but there are a number of books, films and internet resources I must mention here.

Books

K H Denning (ed), *Evidence-based Practice in Dementia for Nurses and Nursing Students*, JKP, 2019. Does what it says on the tin. It is a pretty readable and well-organised study course on dementia.

Annie Dransfield, *Releasing the Compassion,* Amazon, 2021, is a blistering account by a carer who, like me, has been driven into print by the way the system treats (or doesn't) carers and their loved ones.

Frederick Earlstein, *Dementia. Facts and Information*, Amazon, 2016. A quick read though some of the headline topics surrounding dementia.

Lisa Genova, *Still Alice*, Simon and Shuster, 2007. This debut novel by a neuroscientist became hugely popular as an account of Alzheimer's and the way in which it impacted on a leading academic. Worth a read, although I found it a bit stodgy in places. Kleenex required.

Tom Kitwood. *Dementia Reconsidered, revisited. the Person still comes first,* Open University, 2019. This is the second edition, in which Kitwood's text is set against more recent views.

Make sure you get this later edition. A fascinating read, if you want to take up the challenge. There is some technical stuff, but the human and humane qualities of Kitwood and the editor of the new edition, Dawn Brooker, shine through. I had to stop reading the book several times, so poignantly accurate are his observations about patient care.

Wendy Mitchell *Someone I used to know*, Bloomsbury, 2019. A prominent NHS manager works on despite the challenges of dementia. A heart-rending account of one woman's attempts to live on despite her diagnosis. Pass the Kleenex.

Wendy Mitchell, *What I wish people knew about dementia*, Bloomsbury, 2022, is the follow-up to the previous book. More paper handkerchieves to the ready.

Shibley Rhaman and Professor Rob Howard, *Essentials of Dementia*, JKP, 2018. This is a textbook for students, but is nonetheless well worth reading as it is a model of clarity and comprehensiveness.

Films

There are a handful of worthwhile films around on the subject of mental health issues, especially dementia. I have not seen Julianne Moore in *Still Alice* (2014), the film of the novel referred to just now, but I guess it will be worth it just to watch a star actress at work. Alec Baldwin also stars.

There are two British films which Rusalka saw with me way back in the days when dementia was something which happened to other people, not us. The first is *Iris* (2001), another production with two fine actors, Judi Dench and Jim Broadbent. This will just about tug the heartstrings out of you. It's an account of the novelist Iris Murdoch, her younger days and her descent into Alzheimer's. If you see a CD of the musical score in a charity shop, grab it and weep.

Next up is *The Iron Lady* (2011), with Meryl Streep brilliant in the title role, and Jim Broadbent equally as Dennis Thatcher. It explores the contrasts between the past glories and the challenges of dementia. Some reviews were unkind, but Streep as Thatcher steals the show.

Can I also mention *Awakenings* (1990), with Robert de Niro in the lead as a doctor who promotes L-Dopa for the treatment of Parkinsons in catatonic patients who are temporarily revived by the experiment. Sounds dry and technical but it is an extremely sensitive and moving account of mental illness.

Websites

How long have you got? The internet is crawling with sites about dementia in all its manifestations, and many of them duplicate information and advice.

A lot of them are from profit-making organisaions but that doesn't mean they are not to be valued. I was very much impressed by www.completecare.ca. This is a company specialising in dementia care. They do have pages of excellent advice, and I acknowledge that I have exploited some of it in this book.

In the UK, www.carersuk.org website focuses on the needs of carers and is very well worth a visit. There's a well-designed site from www.ageuk.org.uk, but for me top of the list is the Alzheimer's Society website, which has an almost overwhelming amount of quality information on hand. Reach them at www.alzheimers.org.uk.

The Alzheimer's Society has an excellent webpage on the feelings of loss and grief as dementia advances, to be found at https://www.alz.org/help-support/caregiving/caregiver-health/grief-loss-as-alzheimers-progresses.

And finally, for more films on dementia there is a website for them, too:

www.verywellhealth.com/movies-about-dementia-and-alzheimers-disease-97664

This site lists movies on the theme of dementia, but they do come with a gentle reminder that these are above all intended to entertain an audience, so they may not be entirely in line with the facts of dementia, and also they may sideslip the more uncomfortable issues involved.

A clutch of quotes to end with

We remember their love when they can no longer remember. – Alzheimers.net.

One person caring about another represents life's greatest value. – Jim Rohn.

Dementia care—it's not rocket science, it's heart science. – Gail Weatherill, RN.

Release in your mind who your loved one used to be and accept who they are today. – J. Rusnak, PhD.

I like it when people remember that I'm a person, not just a person with Alzheimer's. – Sally Hepworth.

The disease might hide the person underneath, but there's still a person in there who needs your love and attention. – Jamie Calandriello.

You have not lived today until you have done something for someone who can never repay you. – John Bunyan.

Dementia does not rob someone of their dignity. It's our reaction to them that does. – Teepa Snow.

The measure of life isn't its duration, but its donation. – Peter Marshall.

Doctors diagnose, nurses heal and caregivers make sense of it all. – Brett H. Lewis.

In youth we run into difficulties. In old age difficulties run into us. – Josh Billings.

Age is not a particularly interesting subject. Anyone can get old. All you have to do is live long enough. – Groucho Marx.

It's an epitome of life. The first half of it consists of the capacity to enjoy without the chance; the last half consists of the chance without the capacity. – Mark Twain.

If you live to be one hundred, you've got it made. Very few people die past that age. – George Burns.

You're not as young as you used to be. But you're not as old as you're going to be. – Irish saying.

A man who correctly guesses a woman's age may be smart, but he's not very bright. – Lucille Ball.

Children are a great comfort in your old age - and they help you reach it faster, too. – Lionel Kauffman.

I've learned that regardless of color or age, we all need about the same amount of love. – H. Jackson Brown, Jr.

You end up as you deserve. In old age you must put up with the face, the friends, the health, and the children you have earned. – Fay Weldon.

Old age is like a plane flying through a storm. Once you're aboard, there's nothing you can do. – Golda Meir.

Growing old is mandatory; growing up is optional. – Chili Davis.

One of the good things about getting older is you find you're more interesting than most of the people you meet. -- Lee Marvin.

You know you're getting old when you get that one candle on the cake. It's like, 'See if you can blow this out'. – Jerry Seinfeld.

Mother told me there would be days like this, but not so many of them. – 'Bill King'.

Printed in Great Britain
by Amazon